Vegetarian Cookbook For Weigth Loss

A Complete Vegetarian Guide For Weigth Loss And Increase Your Energy

Brigitte S. Romeo

Vegetarian Cookbook For Weigth Loss

© **Copyright 2021 - All rights reserved.**

The content contained within this book may not be reproduced, duplicated or transmitted without direct written permission from the author or the publisher.

Under no circumstances will any blame or legal responsibility be held against the publisher, or author, for any damages, reparation, or monetary loss due to the information contained within this book. Either directly or indirectly.

Legal Notice:

This book is copyright protected. This book is only for personal use. You cannot amend, distribute, sell, use, quote or paraphrase any part, or the content within this book, without the consent of the author or publisher.

Disclaimer Notice:

Please note the information contained within this document is for educational and entertainment purposes only. All effort has been executed to present accurate, up to date, and reliable, complete information. No warranties of any kind are declared or implied. Readers acknowledge that the author is not engaging in the rendering of legal, financial, medical or professional advice. The content within this book has been derived from various sources. Please consult a licensed professional before attempting any techniques outlined in this book.

By reading this document, the reader agrees that under no circumstances is the author responsible for any losses, direct or indirect, which are incurred as a result of the use of information contained within this document, including, but not limited to, errors, omissions, or inaccuracies.

TABLE OF CONTENTS

INTRODUCTION **8**

CHAPTER 1: BREAKFAST RECIPES **12**

1. Spaghetti Squash with Pesto and Fresh Mozzarella 13
2. Speedy Scratch Mac 'n' Cheese 15
3. Steamed Broccoli or Cauliflower, Four Ways 17
4. Steamed Artichokes 19
5. Steamed Asparagus, Four Ways 21
6. Seasoned Bok Choy 23
7. Spicy Kale 25

CHAPTER 2: LUNCH RECIPES **28**

8. Sautéed Collard Greens 28
9. French Fries 30
10. Easy Vegan Pizza Bread 32

CHAPTER 3: MAIN MEALS RECIPES **34**

11. Sweet Potato Tacos 35
12. Marinated Mushroom Scramble 37
13. Mac 'N' Mince 39

CHAPTER 4: VEGETABLES, SALADS AND SIDES RECIPES **42**

14. Flawless Feta and Spinach Pancakes 43
15. Baked Potato Salad 45
16. Tropical Fruit Salad 47
17. Cilantro Lime Coleslaw 48
18. Pesto Pasta Salad 50
19. Veggie Hummus Pinwheels 51
20. Caramelized Onion and Beet Salad 52

21. CORN COBS 54

CHAPTER 5: DESSERT RECIPES 56

22. RASPBERRY LIME SORBET 56
23. BAKED APPLES WITH DRIED FRUIT 58
24. HEMP SEED BRITTLE 60

CHAPTER 6: SNACK RECIPES 62

25. BUTTERMILK PANNA COTTA WITH MANGO 62
26. SWEET POTATO–CINNAMON PARFAITS 65
27. SUN-DRIED TOMATO PESTO SNAPPER 67
28. TROUT-CILANTRO PACKETS 69
29. SOUSED HERRING 71
30. TRADITIONAL SUCCOTASH 73
31. BLACK-EYED PEA KALE BOWL 75

CHAPTER 7: JUICES AND SMOOTHIES RECIPES 78

32. GROOVY GREEN SMOOTHIE 78
33. SUN JUICE 80
34. PROTEIN-PACKED BLUEBERRY SMOOTHIE 81
35. STRAWBERRY PROTEIN SMOOTHIE 82
36. RASPBERRY AVOCADO SMOOTHIE 83
37. EASY ANTIOXIDANT SMOOTHIE 84

CHAPTER 8: OTHER RECIPES 86

38. BLACK BEANS & BROWN RICE 86
39. BEANS & GREENS BOWL 88
40. MILLET AND TEFF WITH SQUASH & ONIONS 89
41. QUESADILLA WITH BLACK BEANS AND SWEET POTATO ... 90
42. MEATLESS CHICK NUGGETS 92
43. APPLE MINT SALAD WITH PINE NUT CRUNCH 94

44.	Pleasant Lemonade	96
45.	Soothing Ginger Tea Drink	97
46.	Nice Spiced Cherry Cider	99
47.	Fragrant Spiced Coffee	101
48.	Banana Chips	103
49.	Dehydrated Oranges	104
50.	Sweet Potato Mash	105

CONCLUSION **108**

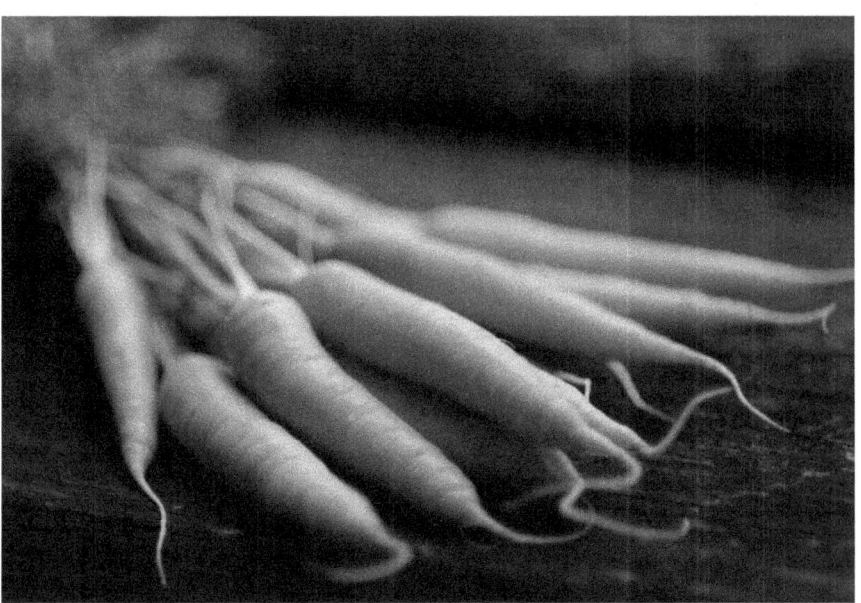

INTRODUCTION

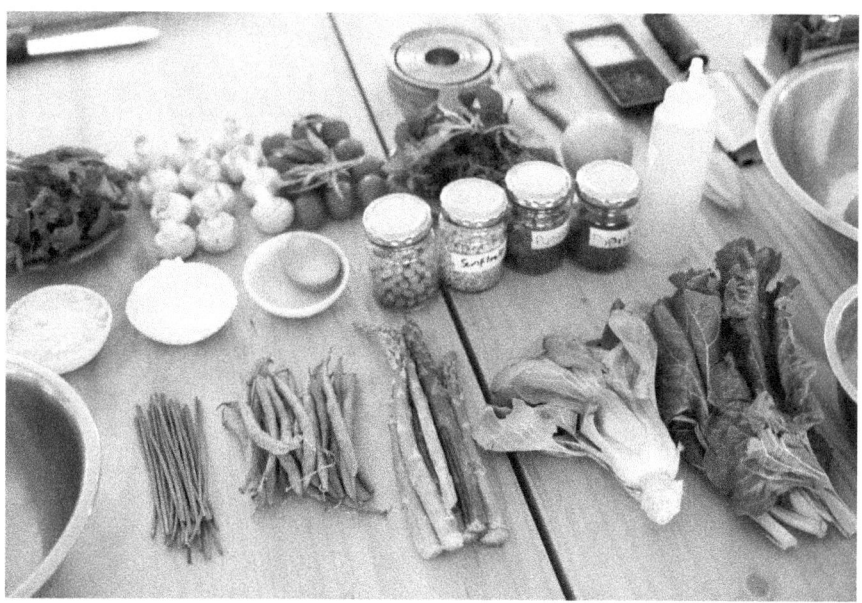

What does it mean to be a vegetarian?

A Vegetarian is a person who does not eat meat, poultry, or fish. Vegetarians eat only plant foods such as fruits, vegetables, legumes, and grains or products made from them. Some people think of a vegetarian as a person who does not eat red meat but may consume fish and chicken. Other people consider a vegetarian to be someone who avoids eating all animal flesh, including fish, poultry, and red meat. However, "true" vegetarians avoid the consumption of all meats, including fish and chicken.

Vegetarianism is not a new concept; it has been practiced since ancient

How often should you eat fruits and vegetables? The recommendation is to eat five servings per day based on a 2,000 calorie diet. One serving is equal to one-half cup raw or one cup ready-to-eat. Fruits and vegetables provide vitamins, minerals, fiber, and other nutrients that are essential for good health. It is recommended that most Americans make fruits and vegetables the basis of their diet; ideally, they should be eaten at every meal.

So, specifically, what are the foods that one needs to avoid? These are as follows:

- Beef
- Pork
- Lamb
- Veal
- All Game (deer, elk, etc.)
- Any other land mammal that's been fed animal products or by-products such as eggs and dairy (many land mammals are herbivores)
- Fish and Shellfish
- Goose and Duck
- Emu and Alligator
- Any other animal that is not a seafood product
- Animal by-products such as gelatin (e.g., gummy bears)

As a vegetarian, what specific foods do you avoid? For starters, you can limit your consumption of the following:

- Pork and bacon
- Eggs (or eat only eggs that are certified organic or non-cage free)

- Dairy products (or consume only dairy products that are certified organic)

- All products that are made from animals, such as leather shoes, belts, jackets, etc.

What are the substitutes that you use to replace the meat and fish that you avoid?

- Tofu (made from soybeans)

- Tempeh (made from soybeans)

- TVP (textured vegetable protein)

- Seitan (very high in protein, available as steak strips or chicken-style pieces)

- Soy Nuggets/Sausage

Being a vegetarian has its benefits, but there are definitely some challenges as well. If you are considering the option of being a vegetarian, the most important thing to consider is your overall health. However, if you have concerns with the lack of protein in your diet, believe that it's unwise to eat only plant products, or simply crave meat and fish and think you can't give them up without feeling hungry or deprived, then the choice of becoming a vegetarian may not be the right one for you.

This vegetarian cookbook will help you get a delicious and healthy recipe on the table that will make your life less stressful. A good recipe doesn't need a long list of ingredients to make it tasty, and while preparing meals may seem hard. You can eat together a healthy family food in the same amount of time you'd need to order takeout!

This vegetarian cookbook will show you a variety of dishes you can make with easy-to-find ingredients. This is the perfect practical guide for anyone looking to make a variety of delicious meals that are healthy. It includes recipes for breakfast, lunch, dinner, appetizers, and desserts, as well as those for snacks and sides. Whether looking to lose weight or just eat more healthily, this cookbook will make it easier than ever before!

So, let us begin the journey.

CHAPTER 1:

BREAKFAST RECIPES

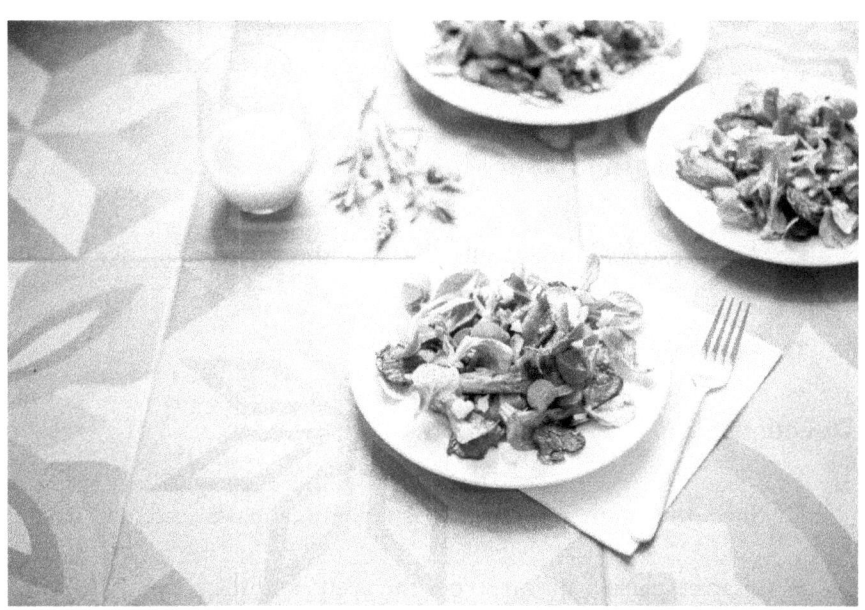

1. Spaghetti Squash with Pesto and Fresh Mozzarella

Preparation Time: 10 minutes

Cooking Time: 7 minutes

Servings: 4

Ingredients:

- 2 (3-pound) spaghetti squash
- 1 cup water
- ½ cup prepared pesto
- 8 ounces fresh mozzarella cheese, cubed
- 2 cups quartered cherry tomatoes

Directions:

1. Slice the stem end of the spaghetti squash and cut it into quarters. Use a spoon to get the seeds and the pulp.
2. Place a rack or a steamer insert in the pressure cooker pot and add the water to the pot. Place the squash on the rack or steamer, cut-side down. The squash can be layered on top of

each other, but shouldn't fill the pot more than two-thirds full. If it doesn't all fit, cook it in two batches.

3. Lock lid and set the timer for 7 minutes at high pressure. When the timer is off, quick release the pressure, open the cooker, and remove the squash with tongs.

4. If squash is cool enough to handle, use a fork to scrape the squash into strands, transferring them to a large bowl. Spoon the pesto over the squash, and use tongs to toss the squash, distributing the pesto to evenly coat the squash. Add the mozzarella and cherry tomatoes, and toss to combine. Serve warm or at room temperature.

Nutrition: Calories: 190 Carbs: 12g Fat: 10g Protein: 12g

2. Speedy Scratch Mac 'n' Cheese

Preparation Time: 10 minutes

Cooking Time: 5 minutes

Servings: 4

Ingredients:

- 8 ounces elbow macaroni
- 1 cup evaporated milk, divided
- 1¼ cups water
- 1½ teaspoons kosher salt
- 1 teaspoon dried mustard
- 1 egg
- 8 ounces extra-sharp Cheddar cheese, grated
- 1½ teaspoons cornstarch

Directions:

1. In the pot pressure cooker, add the macaroni, ¾ cup of evaporated milk, water, salt, and dried mustard. Stir to combine.

2. Lock lid and set the timer for 5 minutes at high pressure.

3. Meanwhile, in a small bowl, whisk the egg. Add ¼ cup of evaporated milk and whisk to combine.

4. Place the grated cheese in a medium bowl and sprinkle the cornstarch over the cheese. Toss to coat.

5. When the pressure cooker timer goes off, quick release the pressure. Test the macaroni, if it is not quite done, switch the setting to sauté or brown, and simmer it for 1 to 2 minutes, covered, until tender.

6. If you haven't switched the setting, switch the setting to sauté or brown and add the milk-egg mixture and a large handful of cheese. Stir to melt the cheese. Continue adding the cheese in several handfuls, stirring until it completely melts with each addition. Serve immediately.

Nutrition: Calories: 367 Carbs: 40g Fat: 16g Protein: 13g

3. Steamed Broccoli or Cauliflower, Four Ways

Preparation Time: 10 minutes

Cooking Time: 2 minutes

Servings: 4

Ingredients:

- 1 broccoli head, cut into bite-size florets (about 4 cups) or 1 cauliflower head, cut into bite-size florets (about 4 cups)
- 1 tablespoon extra-virgin olive oil
- 2 tablespoons melted unsalted butter
- ¼ cup toasted bread crumbs
- 2 tablespoons balsamic vinaigrette
- 2 tablespoons grated parmesan cheese
- Salt and pepper

Directions:

1. Place a steamer insert in the pot of a pressure cooker. Add the water to the pot. Place the broccoli or cauliflower in the insert.

2. Lock lid and set the timer for 2 minutes at high pressure. When the timer is off, quick release the pressure and open the lid. Use tongs to transfer the broccoli or cauliflower to a serving dish.

3. Top or toss broccoli with one of the following:

4. 2 tablespoons melted unsalted butter and ¼ cup toasted bread crumbs that have been mixed with 2 tablespoons grated Parmesan cheese. Season with salt and pepper.

5. 1 tablespoon extra-virgin olive oil and ¼ cup crumbled feta or goat cheese. Season with salt and pepper.

6. 1 tablespoon extra-virgin olive oil. Then sprinkle it with red pepper flakes, salt, and pepper.

7. 2 tablespoons prepared or homemade balsamic vinaigrette

Nutrition: Calories: 68 Carbs: 9g Fat: 3g Protein: 1g

4. **Steamed Artichokes**

Preparation Time: 10 minutes

Cooking Time: 15 minutes

Servings: 4

Ingredients:

- 4 medium artichokes
- 1 lemon, halved
- 1 cup water

Directions:

1. To prepare the artichokes, use kitchen shears to trim the spiky tips off all the artichoke leaves. Pull any tough leaves off the very bottom and use a paring knife to trim off the stem. Rub cut parts of the artichoke with the lemon to avoid discoloring.

2. Place a steamer insert or a rack in the pressure cooker pot.

3. Add the water to the pot. Arrange the artichokes in the pressure cooker, stacking them if necessary.

4. Lock lid and set the timer for 15 minutes at high pressure. When the timer is off, quick release the pressure, open the lid, and remove the artichokes with tongs. Serve hot or cool or use in another recipe.

Nutrition: Calories: 27 Carbs: 6g Fat: 0g Protein: 2g

5. Steamed Asparagus, Four Ways

Preparation Time: 5 minutes

Cooking Time: 1 minute

Servings: 4

Ingredients:

- ½ cup water
- 1 pound asparagus, trimmed
- 2 tablespoons melted unsalted butter mixed
- ½ teaspoon freshly grated lemon zest
- 2 tablespoons champagne vinaigrette
- 1 tablespoon slivered almonds
- ¼ cup hollandaise sauce
- 1 tablespoon hazelnut oil
- 1 tablespoon chopped hazelnuts
- Salt and pepper

Directions:

1. Place a steamer insert in the pot of a pressure cooker. Add the water to the pot. Place the asparagus in the insert. If the stalks are too long, it's fine to lean them against the sides of the cooker.

2. Lock the lid and then set the timer for 1 minute at high pressure. When the timer is off, quick release the pressure and open the lid. Transfer the asparagus to a plate.

3. Top or toss asparagus with one of the following:

4. 2 tablespoons melted unsalted butter mixed with ½ teaspoon freshly grated lemon zest

5. 2 tablespoons champagne vinaigrette and 1 tablespoon slivered almonds

6. ¼ cup hollandaise sauce

7. 1 tablespoon hazelnut oil and 1 tablespoon chopped hazelnuts. Season with salt and pepper.

Nutrition: Calories: 32 Carbs: 3g Fat: 1g Protein: 5g

6. Seasoned Bok Choy

Preparation Time: 5 minutes

Cooking Time: 1 minute

Servings: 4

Ingredients:

- 1 cup water
- 4 baby bok choy heads, quartered lengthwise
- 1 tablespoon rice wine vinegar
- 1 teaspoon sesame oil
- 1 tablespoon toasted sesame seeds

Directions:

1. Place a steamer insert in the pot of a pressure cooker. Add the water to the cooker and mound the bok choy in the steamer.
2. Lock lid and set the timer for 1 minute at high pressure. When the timer is off, quick release the pressure and remove the cover, transfer the bok choy to the platter or bowl.

3. In the bowl, whisk together the vinegar and sesame oil. Drizzle it over the bok choy. Sprinkle the sesame seeds over the bok choy and serve immediately.

Nutrition: Calories: 13 Carbs: 2g Fat: 0g Protein: 2g

7. Spicy Kale

Preparation Time: 1 minute

Cooking Time: 5 minutes

Servings: 4

Ingredients:

- 1 tablespoon extra-virgin olive oil
- 2 garlic cloves, minced
- 1 kale bunch, stemmed and chopped or 1 (1-pound) bag chopped kale
- 1½ cups water
- 1 tablespoon red wine vinegar
- ½ teaspoon red pepper flakes
- ¼ teaspoon kosher salt

Directions:

1. With the pressure cooker on the sauté or brown setting, heat the olive oil. Add the garlic and sauté for 30 seconds, stirring constantly. Add the kale and water to the pressure cooker.

2. Then lock the lid and set the timer for 5 minutes at high pressure. When the timer is off, quick release the pressure, remove the lid, and toss the cooked greens with the vinegar, red pepper flakes, and salt. Serve hot.

Nutrition: Calories: 65 Carbs: 1g Fat: 1g Protein: 1g

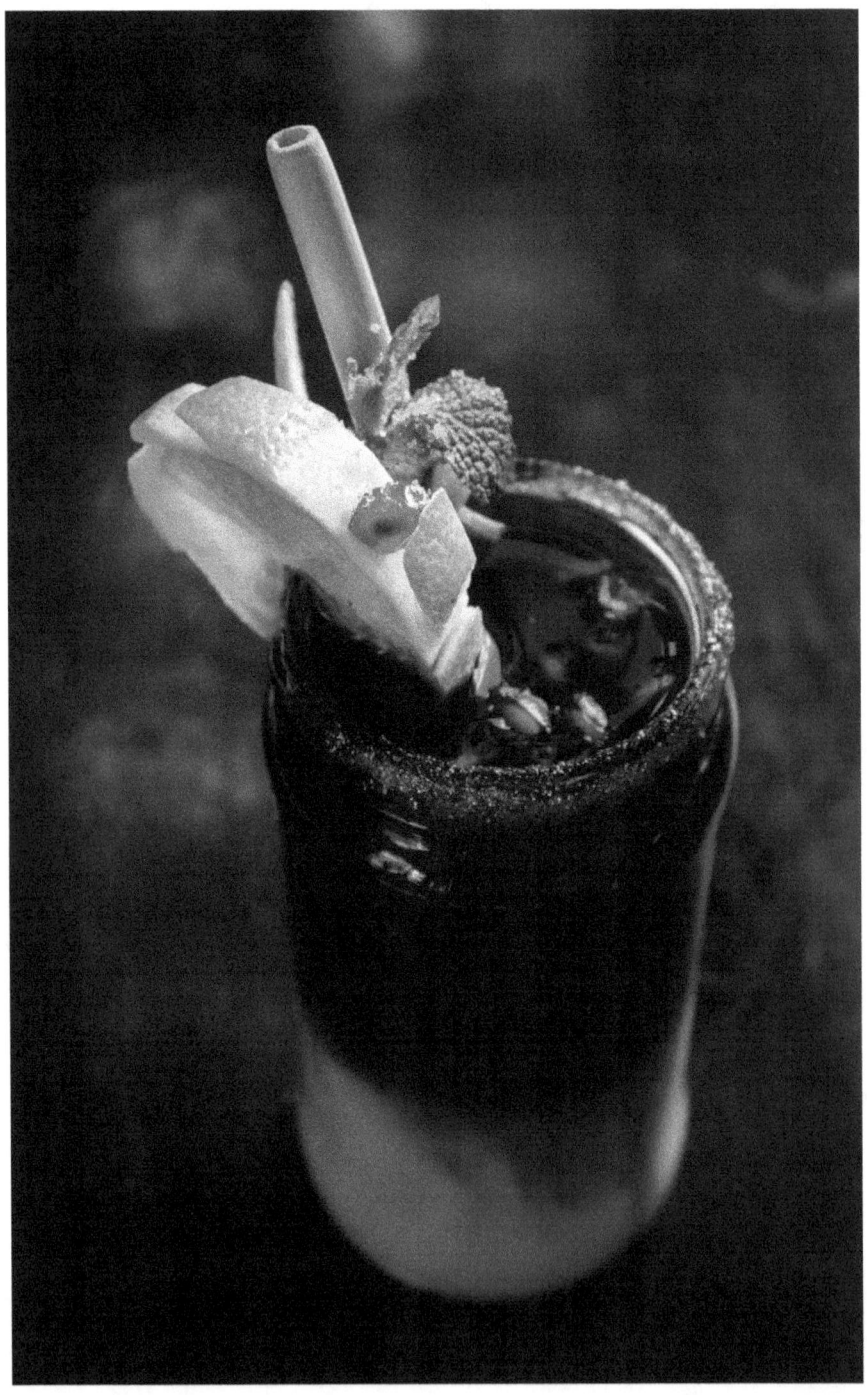

CHAPTER 2:

LUNCH RECIPES

8. Sautéed Collard Greens

Preparation Time: 10 minutes

Cooking Time: 25 minutes

Servings: 4

Ingredients:

- 1½ pounds collard greens

- 1 cup vegetable broth

- ½ teaspoon garlic powder

- ½ teaspoon onion powder

- ⅛ teaspoon freshly ground black pepper

Directions:

1. Remove the hard middle stems from the greens, then roughly chop the leaves into 2-inch pieces.

2. In a large saucepan, mix together the vegetable broth, garlic powder, onion powder, and pepper. Bring to a boil over medium-high heat, then add the chopped greens. Reduce the heat to low and cover.

3. Cook for 20 minutes, stirring well every 4 to 5 minutes, and serve.

Nutrition: Calories: 28 Total fat: 1g Carbohydrates: 4g Fiber: 2g Protein: 3g

9. French Fries

Preparation Time: 10 minutes

Cooking Time: 60 minutes

Servings: 6

Ingredients:

- 2 pounds medium white potatoes

- 1 to 2 tablespoons no-salt seasoning

Directions:

1. Preheat the oven to 400°F. Line a baking sheet with parchment paper.

2. Wash and scrub potatoes and place them on the baking sheet and bake for 45 minutes.

3. Remove potatoes from the oven. Allow to cool in the refrigerator for about 30 minutes, or until you're ready to make a batch of fries.

4. Preheat the oven to 425°F. Line a baking sheet with parchment paper.

5. Slice the cooled potatoes into the shape of wedges or fries, then toss them in a large bowl with the no-salt seasoning.

6. Spread the coated fries out in an even layer on the baking sheet. Bake for about 7 minutes, then remove from the oven, flip the fries over, and redistribute them in an even layer. Bake again for another 8 minutes, or until the fries are crisp and golden brown, and serve.

Nutrition: Calories: 104 Total fat: 0g Carbohydrates: 24g Fiber: 4g Protein: 3g

10. Easy Vegan Pizza Bread

Preparation Time: 5 minutes Cooking Time: 20 minutes

Servings: 4

Ingredients:

- 1 whole-wheat loaf, unsliced
- 1 cup Easy One-Pot Vegan Marinara
- 1 teaspoon nutritional yeast
- ½ teaspoon onion powder
- ½ teaspoon garlic powder

Directions:

1. Preheat the oven to 375°F. Halve the loaf of bread lengthwise. Evenly spread the marinara onto each slice of bread, then sprinkle on the nutritional yeast, onion powder, and garlic powder. Place bread on a baking sheet. Bake for 20 minutes, or until the bread is a light golden brown.

Nutrition: Calories: 230 Total fat: 3g Carbohydrates: 38g Fiber: 7g Protein: 13g

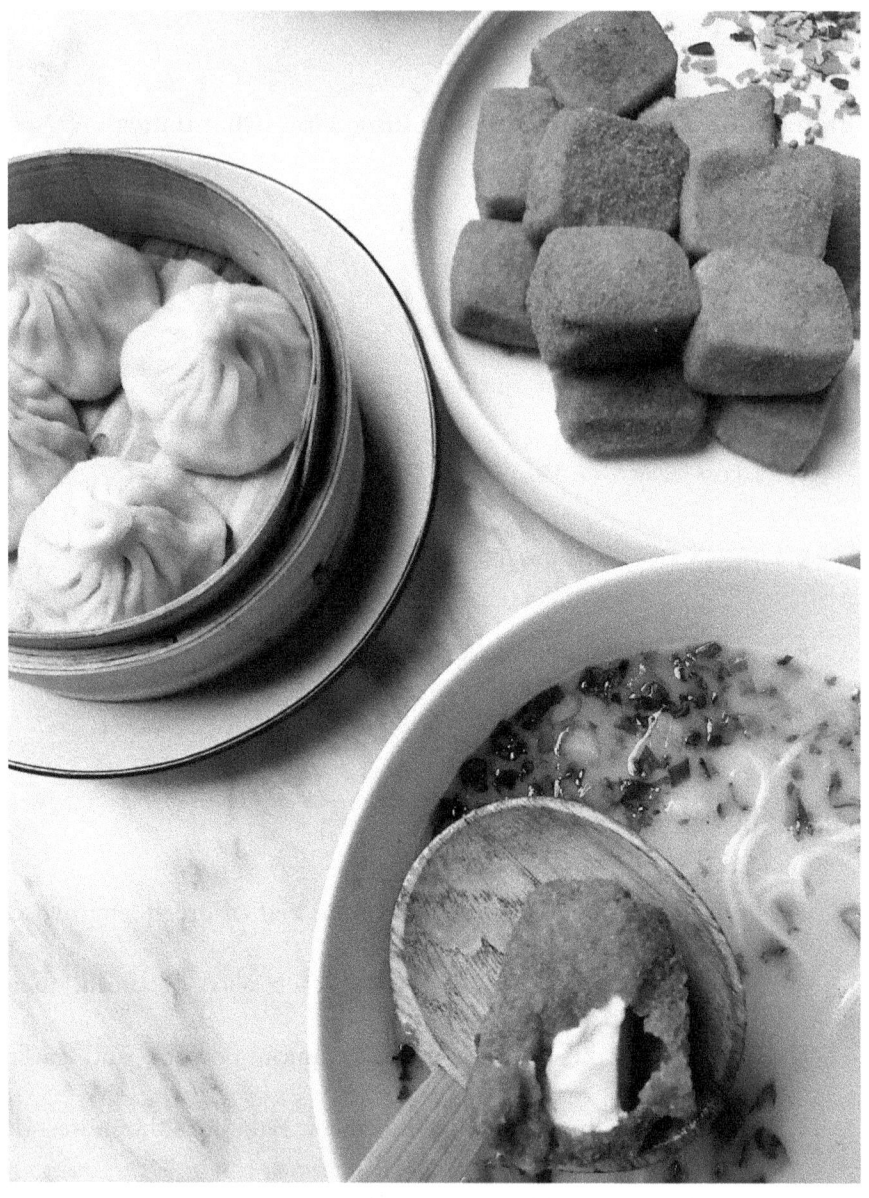

CHAPTER 3:

MAIN MEALS RECIPES

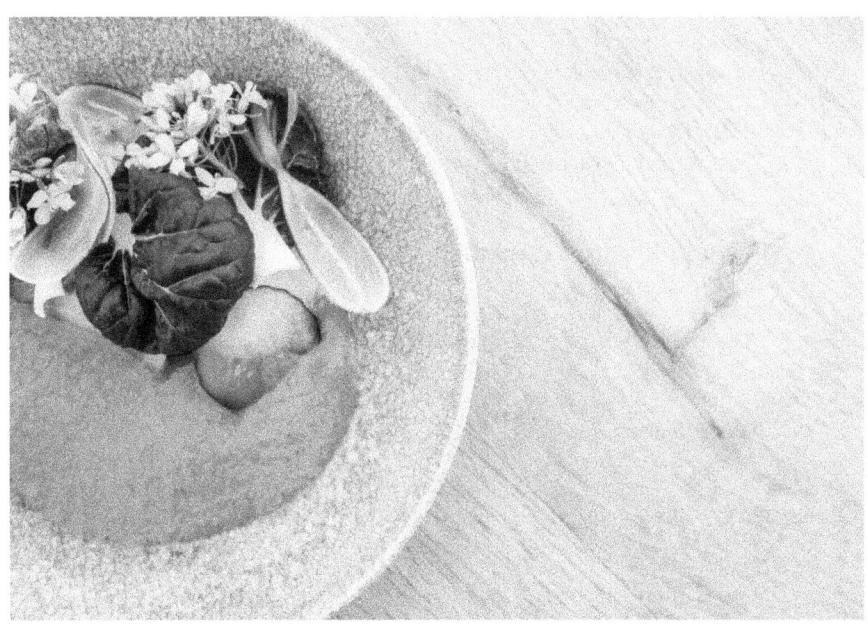

11. Sweet Potato Tacos

Preparation Time: 15 minutes

Cooking Time: 5 minutes

Servings: 6

Ingredients:

- 2 cups Black beans (cooked or canned)
- 1 7-oz pack textured soy mince
- 3 small sweet potatoes (cubed)
- 6 whole wheat taco shells
- ¼ cup Mexican chorizo seasoning
- 1 cup Water

Directions:

1. When using dry beans, soak and cook 1½ cup (113 g.) of dry black beans according to the procedure.

2. Put water in a pot, then put cubed potatoes. Make sure to pot is over medium-high heat for 15 minutes or until cooked. Drain excess water, then set aside the potatoes.

3. Put the pan over medium-high heat. Make sure to use a non-stick pan. Add soy mince, black beans, chorizo seasoning, and a cup of water.

4. Stir continuously until everything is cooked, then add the cooked sweet potato cubes.

5. Turn the heat off, then stir occasionally for 5 minutes until cooked.

6. Divide sweet potato mixture for 6 taco shells.

7. Serve and enjoy!

Nutrition: Calories: 202 Carbs: 29.7 g. Fat: 2.85 g. Protein: 13.2 g.

12. Marinated Mushroom Scramble

Preparation Time: 15 minutes

Cooking Time: 15 minutes

Servings: 4

Ingredients:

- 2 cups Button mushrooms
- 1 14-ounces pack Extra-firm tofu (scrambled)
- 2 medium yellow onions (thinly sliced)
- ¼ cup Low-sodium soy sauce
- ½ cup Tahini
- ½ cup Water

Directions:

1. Add the mushrooms, tofu scramble, and soy sauce to an airtight container.

2. Then close the lid and shake well until everything is evenly covered with soy sauce.

3. Put the container in the fridge and leave to marinate for at least an hour or up to 12 hours.

4. Put the pan over medium heat. Add the water and tofu mushroom mixture to the pan.

5. Add onion, then cook it for 15 minutes, stirring occasionally with a spatula to prevent the tofu from sticking to the pan, until the mushrooms are cooked, and most of the water has evaporated.

6. Turn the heat off and divide tofu mushroom scramble into 2 bowls.

7. Top the bowls with the tahini, serve with the optional toppings, and enjoy!

8. Store the tofu mushroom scramble in an airtight container in the fridge.

Nutrition: Calories: 340 Carbs: 12.6 g. Fat: 23.3 g. Protein: 20 g.

13. Mac 'N' Mince

Preparation Time: 15 minutes

Cooking Time: 10 minutes

Servings: 4

Ingredients:

- 2 cups Whole wheat macaroni
- 7-ounces pack textured soy mince
- ½ cup Tahini
- ¼ cup Nutritional yeast
- 2 tablespoons Lemon garlic pepper seasoning
- ½ cup Water

Directions:

1. Cook the macaroni according to instructions and then set it aside afterward.

2. Put a frying pan over medium-high heat. Make sure to use a non-stick pan, then add the soy mince together with the ¼ cup water.

3. Stir fry soy mince until cooked and make sure most of the water evaporated.

4. Then add the ¼ cup of water, nutritional yeast, lemon garlic pepper seasoning, tahini, and then put turmeric to the soy mince, but this is optional.

5. Cook a little longer until well combined.

6. Add the cooked macaroni to the pan with soy mince. Stir this thoroughly until mixed well.

7. Divide mac 'n' mince into two plates. Serve and enjoy!

Nutrition: Calories: 454 Carbs: 42 g. Fat: 19.9 g. Protein: 25.05 g

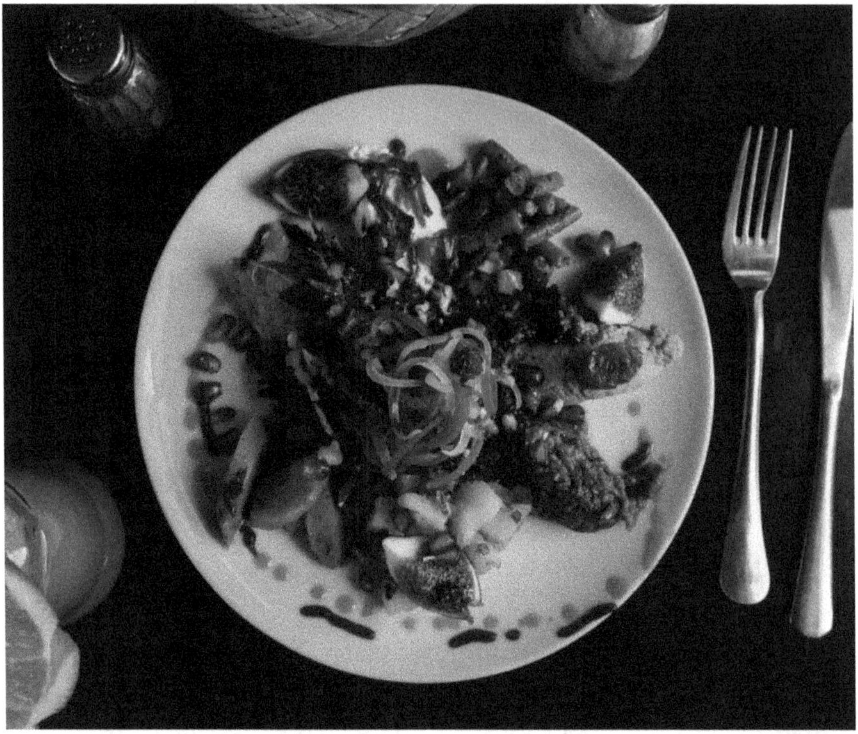

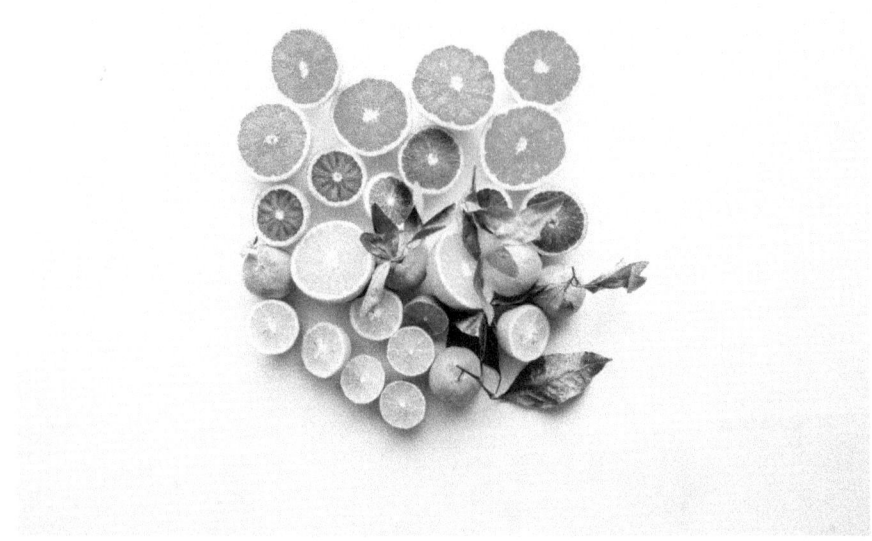

CHAPTER 4:

VEGETABLES, SALADS AND SIDES RECIPES

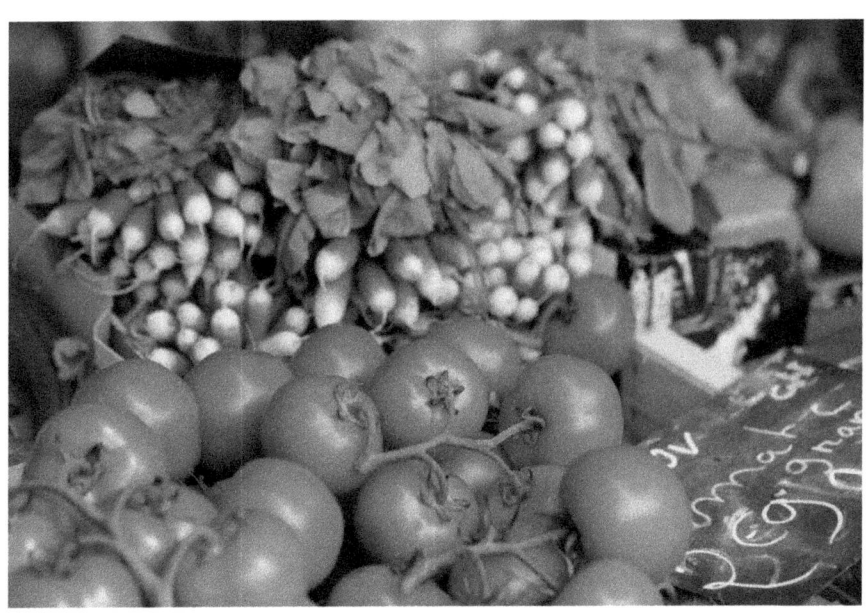

14. Flawless Feta and Spinach Pancakes

Preparation Time: 10 minutes

Cooking Time: 20 minutes

Servings: 4

Ingredients:

- 17 ounces spinach, frozen
- 1 cup flour
- 2 eggs
- 1 cup milk
- 5 ounces feta cheese

What you'll need from the store cupboard

- 2 tablespoons butter
- Salt to taste

Directions:

1. Heat a pot on and put it in medium heat. Add the frozen spinach. Stir frequently to deforest the spinach quickly.

2. Add flour, eggs, and milk in a mixing bowl, then use a hand mixer to mix until there are no lumps.

3. Add more milk until consistency is achieved.

4. Heat a nonstick skillet over medium heat.

5. Melt butter and pour the mixture into the pan — Fry for four minutes on each side.

6. Layer the pancake on a plate, then pour the heated spinach on one half of the pancake.

7. Layer cheese slices on the spinach, then fold the pancake. Serve and enjoy.

Nutrition: Calories 361 Fat 18g Carbs 33g Protein 17g

15. Baked Potato Salad

Preparation Time: 10 minutes

Cooking Time: 30 minutes

Servings: 6-8

Ingredients:

- 6 cups cooked potatoes cut into slices
- 1 cup chopped celery
- ⅔ cup brown sugar
- ⅔ cup vinegar
- 1 ⅓ cup water
- Olive oil for cooking

Directions:

1. Preheat the oven to 350 F.
2. Pour an amount of olive oil into the frying pan and turn the heat to medium. Lightly sauté the celery.
3. Add the sugar, vinegar, and water and bring to a boil. Adjust the heat on low and let simmer for 5 minutes.

4. Fill your oven dish with the cooked potato and pour the vinegar sauce over. Make sure the potatoes are completely covered.

5. Bake the potatoes for about 20 minutes in the oven.

6. This dish works both warm and cold.

Nutrition: Calories 250 Fat 19g Carbs 18g Protein 4g

16. Tropical Fruit Salad

Preparation Time: 10 minutes

Cooking Time: 0 minutes

Servings: 2

Ingredients:

- 1 cup of dragon fruit
- 1 cup ripe mango
- 1 tablespoon lime juice
- 12 Strawberries
- 2 Kiwis

Directions:

1. Peel all of the fruits and then chop them into small, bite-sized pieces. Dump all of the chunks of fruit into a large-sized mixing bowl. Drizzle the lime juice over the fruit and toss the fruit gently to coat all of the pieces with the juice. Serve immediately

Nutrition: Calories 154 Fat 1g Carbs 37g Protein 3g

17. Cilantro Lime Coleslaw

Preparation Time: 10 minutes

Cooking Time: 0 minutes

Servings: 5

Ingredients:

- 2 pieces of avocados
- 1 tablespoon garlic, minced
- 14 ounces coleslaw
- ¼ cilantro, fresh leaves, minced
- 2 tablespoons lime juice
- ½ teaspoon salt
- ¼ cup water

Directions:

1. Except for the slaw mix, put all of the ingredients that are listed into a blender. Blend these ingredients well until they are creamy and smooth. Mix the coleslaw mix in with this dressing and then toss it gently to mix it well. Keep the mixed coleslaw in the

refrigerator until you are ready to serve. It needs to chill for at least one hour.

Nutrition: Calories 119 Fat 9g Carbs 3g Protein 3g

18. Pesto Pasta Salad

Preparation Time: 5 minutes

Cooking Time: 10 minutes

Servings: 2

Ingredients:

- Fusilli pasta, whole wheat, two cups
- Pesto, low fat, four tablespoons
- Spinach, one cup
- Salt, one half teaspoon
- Black pepper, one half teaspoon

Directions:

1. Cook the fusilli, letting it get slightly overcooked so it will not be sticky when it is cold. Before draining the pasta, drop in the spinach and let it wilt for two to three minutes. Drain the water off the pasta and spinach and pour it into a bowl. Add the pesto, pepper, and salt and mix everything together well.

Nutrition: Calories 340 Fat 2g Carbs 66g Protein 10g

19. Veggie Hummus Pinwheels

Preparation Time: 10 minutes Cooking Time: 0 minutes

Servings: 3

Ingredients:

- 3 whole-grain, spinach, flour, or gluten-free tortillas
- 3 large Swiss chard leaves
- ¾ cup Edamame Hummus or prepared hummus
- ¾ cup shredded carrots

Directions:

1. Lay 1 tortilla flat on a cutting board. Place 1 Swiss chard leaf over the tortilla. Spread ¼ cup of hummus over the Swiss chard. Spread ¼ cup of carrots over the hummus.

2. Starting at one end of the tortilla, roll tightly toward the opposite side. Slice each roll up into 6 pieces. Place in a single-serving storage container. Repeat with the remaining tortillas and filling and seal the lids.

Nutrition: Calories 254 Fat 2g Carbs 39g Protein 10g

20. Caramelized Onion and Beet Salad

Preparation Time: 10 minutes

Cooking Time: 40 minutes

Servings: 4

Ingredients:

- 3 medium golden beets
- 2 cups sliced sweet or Vidalia onions
- 1 teaspoon extra-virgin olive oil or no-beef broth
- Pinch baking soda
- ¼ to ½ teaspoon salt, to taste
- 2 tablespoons unseasoned rice vinegar, white wine vinegar, or balsamic vinegar

Directions:

1. Cut the greens off the beets and scrub the beets. In a large pot, place a steamer basket and fill the pot with 2 inches of water. Add the beets, bring to a boil, then reduce the heat to medium,

cover, and steam for about 35 minutes, until you can easily pierce the middle of the beets with a knife.

2. Meanwhile, in a large, dry skillet over medium heat, sauté the onions for 5 minutes, stirring frequently. Add the olive oil and baking soda, and continuing cooking for 5 more minutes, stirring frequently. Stir in the salt to taste before removing it from the heat. Transfer to a large bowl and set aside.

3. When the beets have cooked through, drain and cool until easy to handle. Rub the beets in a paper towel to easily remove the skins. Cut into wedges, and transfer to the bowl with the onions. Drizzle the vinegar over everything and toss well.

4. Divide the beets evenly among 4 wide-mouth jars or storage containers. Let cool before sealing the lids.

Nutrition: Calories 104 Fat 2g Carbs 20g Protein 3g

21. Corn Cobs

Preparation Time: 10 minutes

Cooking Time: 2 minutes

Servings: 4

Ingredients:

- 4 ears corn
- 2 cups water
- Salt and pepper to taste
- 1 tablespoon lemon juice
- 1 tablespoon melted butter

Directions:

1. Add water and arrange the corn ears vertically in the Instant Pot.
2. Keep the larger end of the corn ears dipped in the water or arrange diagonally.
3. Make sure that the lid is closed tightly and select the "Manual" function with high pressure for 2 minutes.

4. After the beep, do a Natural release, then remove the lid carefully?

5. Strain the corn ears and transfer them to a platter.

6. Drizzle some lemon juice along with melted butter on top.

7. Sprinkle salt and pepper, then serve hot.

Nutrition: Calories: 158 Carbohydrate: 29.1g Protein: 5.1g Fat: 4.7g

CHAPTER 5:

DESSERT RECIPES

22. Raspberry Lime Sorbet

Preparation Time: 15 minutes, plus 5 hours or more to chill

Cooking Time: 0 minutes

Servings: 4

Ingredients:

- 3 pints fresh raspberries or 2 (10-ounce) bags frozen
- ½ cup fresh orange juice
- 4 tablespoons pure maple syrup
- 3 tablespoons fresh lime juice
- Dark chocolate curls, optional

Directions:

1. In a glass dish, combine the raspberries, orange juice, maple syrup, and lime juice. Stir well to mix. Cover then put in the freezer until frozen solid, about 5 hours.

2. Get it from the freezer and let it sit for 10 minutes. Crush chunks with a knife or large spoon and transfer the mixture to a food processor. Process this until smooth and creamy for 5 minutes. Serve immediately. The sorbet will freeze solid again, but can be processed again until creamy just before serving.

3. To serve, place a scoop into an ice cream dish. Garnish with fresh raspberries and dark chocolate curls, if using.

4. Preparation Tip: To make chocolate curls, use a vegetable peeler, and scrape the blade lengthwise across a piece of solid chocolate to create pretty, delicate curls. Refrigerate the curls until ready to use.

Nutrition: Calories: 191 Fat: 2g Carbohydrate: 46g Protein: 3g

23. Baked Apples with Dried Fruit

Preparation Time: 10 minutes

Cooking Time: 1 hour

Servings: 4

Ingredients:

- 4 large apples, cored to make a cavity
- 4 teaspoons raisins or cranberries
- 4 teaspoons pure maple syrup
- ½ teaspoon ground cinnamon
- ½ cup unsweetened apple juice or water

Directions:

1. Preheat the oven to 350°F.
2. Place apples in a baking pan that will hold them upright. Put the dried fruit into the cavities and drizzle with maple syrup. Sprinkle with cinnamon. Pour apple juice or water on the apples.
3. Cover loosely with foil and bake for 50 minutes to 1 hour, or until the apples are tender when pierced with a fork.

4. Serving Suggestion: Serve the apples topped with Vegan Whipped Cream.

Nutrition: Calories: 158 Fat: 1g Carbohydrate: 42g Protein: 1g

24. Hemp Seed Brittle

Preparation Time: 10 minutes

Cooking Time: 10 minutes

Servings: 6

Ingredients:

- ¼ cup hemp seeds
- 2½ tablespoons brown rice flour
- 3 tablespoons melted coconut oil
- 2½ tablespoons pure maple syrup
- Pinch salt

Direction:

1. Preheat the oven to 350°F. Line a baking sheet with parchment paper.
2. In a bowl, combine all ingredients, then mix well. Spread into an even layer on the baking sheet. Try to quickly else edges will burn.

3. Bake for 10 minutes and make sure the brittle doesn't burn. Turn off the oven and leave it for 30 minutes to cool down.

4. When it's completely cooled, break it into bite-size pieces with a sharp knife or your fingers.

5. Leftovers: Store leftovers in a sealed container at room temperature for 5 days or freeze for up to 1 month.

Nutrition: Calories: 151 Fat: 12g Carbohydrate: 9g Protein: 4g

CHAPTER 6:

SNACK RECIPES

25. Buttermilk Panna Cotta with Mango

Preparation Time: 10 minutes

Cooking Time: 2 minutes

Servings: 4

Ingredients:

- ½ cup full-fat coconut milk

- 1½ teaspoons agar-agar

- 1½ cups buttermilk

- ¼ cup honey

- 2 cups roughly chopped fresh mango

Directions:

1. Pour coconut milk into a saucepan, then sprinkle the agar-agar over it and let the coconut milk stand for 5 minutes.

2. Put the saucepan over medium-low heat until the agar-agar is dissolved, about 2 minutes.

3. Add the buttermilk and honey and stir to combine.

4. Pour the panna cotta mixture into 4 (6-ounce) ramekins. Wrap it in plastic wrap, then refrigerate them for about 3 hours, or until set.

5. Loosen the panna cotta by running a knife around the inside edges of the ramekins. Invert them onto serving plates.

6. Top with mango and serve.

7. Flavor Boost Vanilla beans add intense flavor and a pretty speckled appearance to this creamy dessert. Cut the vanilla bean in lengthwise and use a paring knife to scrape the seeds from one half into the buttermilk and honey in step 3.

8. Wrap the other vanilla bean half in plastic and store in the fridge to use in smoothies or another dessert.

Nutrition: Calories: 226 Total Fat: 8g Protein: 6g Cholesterol: 4mg Sodium: 106mg Carbohydrates: 36g Fiber: 2g

26. Sweet Potato–Cinnamon Parfaits

Preparation Time: 15 minutes

Cooking Time: 15 minutes

Servings: 4

Ingredients:

- 2 sweet potatoes, cut into ½-inch chunks
- 1 cup coconut cream, chilled in the refrigerator overnight
- ¼ cup maple syrup
- ¼ teaspoon ground cinnamon
- Pinch sea salt
- ½ cup roughly chopped hazelnuts

Directions:

1. Get a large saucepan, then put the sweet potatoes. Fill the pan with water until the sweet potatoes are covered by about an inch. Boil over high heat and then reduce the heat and simmer until sweet potatoes are tender, about 15 minutes. Drain the water and mash sweet potatoes until smooth using a potato masher.

2. Transfer the sweet potatoes to a resealable container, and set it in the refrigerator until completely cooled, about 2 hours.

3. Whip the cold coconut cream until stiff peaks form using a large bowl.Mix the sweet potatoes, maple syrup, cinnamon, and salt, then stir together in a bowl until smooth.

4. Fold half the whipped coconut cream into the sweet potato mixture, keeping as much volume as possible.

5. Chill the sweet potato mixture in the refrigerator for 1 hour.

6. Spoon the sweet potato mixture into 4 bowls and divide the remaining whipped coconut cream between the bowls.

7. Top with hazelnuts before serving.

8. Flavor Boost Hazelnuts have a wonderful, almost buttery-sweet flavor that is enhanced when roasted. Place ½ cup whole hazelnuts on a baking sheet and roast them in a 300°F oven for 10 to 15 minutes. Wait until the nuts cool and rub them between your hands to remove the skins. Chop and store the nuts in a sealed container in the cupboard for up to 1 week.

Nutrition: Calories: 296 Total Fat: 12g Protein: 2g Cholesterol: 0mg Sodium: 70mg Carbohydrates: 41g Fiber: 1g

27. Sun-dried Tomato Pesto Snapper

Preparation Time: 5 minutes

Cooking Time: 15 minutes

Servings: 4

Ingredients:

- 1 sweet onion, cut into ¼-inch slices
- 4 (5-ounce) snapper fillets
- Freshly ground black pepper, for seasoning
- ¼ cup sun-dried tomato pesto
- 2 tablespoons finely chopped fresh basil

Directions:

1. Preheat the oven to 400°F. Put parchment paper in a baking dish and arrange the onion slices on the bottom.
2. Pat the snapper fillets dry with a paper towel and season them lightly with pepper.
3. Place the fillets on the onions and spread 1 tablespoon of pesto on each fillet.

4. Bake until the fish flakes easily with a fork, 12 to 15 minutes.

5. Serve topped with basil.

Nutrition: Calories: 199 Total Fat: 3g Protein: 36g Cholesterol: 66mg Sodium: 119mg Carbohydrates: 3g Fiber: 1g

28. Trout-Cilantro Packets

Preparation Time: 5 minutes

Cooking Time: 20 minutes

Servings: 4

Ingredients:

- 4 cups cauliflower florets
- 2 red bell peppers
- 2 cups snow peas, stringed
- 4 (5-ounce) trout fillets
- Sea salt, for seasoning
- Freshly ground black pepper, for seasoning
- 2 tablespoons olive oil
- 2 tablespoons finely chopped cilantro

Directions:

1. Preheat the oven to 400°F.
2. Prepare four pieces of aluminum foil, each 12 inches square.

3. Evenly divide the cauliflower, bell peppers, and snow peas between the pieces of foil.

4. Pat dry the trout fillets with paper towels. Season them with salt and pepper.

5. Place a fillet on each foil square and drizzle the olive oil over the fish.

6. Fold the foil up to form tightly sealed packets and put them on a baking sheet.

7. Bake until cooked for about 20 minutes.

8. Serve topped with cilantro.

Nutrition: Calories: 398 Total Fat: 23g Saturated Fat: 5g Protein: 35g Cholesterol: 80mg Sodium: 153mg Carbohydrates: 16g Fiber: 6g

29. Soused Herring

Preparation Time: 10 minutes

Cooking Time: 30 minutes

Servings: 4

Ingredients:

- 4 whole herring fillets, scaled, filleted, and trimmed
- 2 cups water
- ½ sweet onion, thinly sliced
- ½ cup white vinegar
- 2 thyme sprigs
- 1 tablespoon granulated sugar
- 1 teaspoon sea salt
- ¼ teaspoon black peppercorns

Directions:

1. Preheat the oven to 350°F.
2. Place the herring fillets in a 9-by-13-inch baking dish.

3. Add the water, onion, white vinegar, thyme, sugar, salt, and peppercorns.

4. Cover baking dish with foil. Bake the fish until tender for 25 to 30 minutes.

5. Cool before serving. This can be stored resealable container for 1 week.

Nutrition: Calories: 277 Total Fat: 15g Protein: 29g Cholesterol: 96mg Sodium: 482mg Carbohydrates: 5g; Fiber: 15g

30. Traditional Succotash

Preparation Time: 10 minutes

Cooking Time: 20 minutes

Servings: 4

Ingredients:

- 2 tablespoons olive oil
- 1 sweet onion, finely chopped
- 1 tablespoon minced garlic
- 2 (15-ounce) cans diced sodium-free tomatoes, undrained
- 2 cups shelled edamame
- 2 cups corn
- 1 orange bell pepper, seeded and diced
- Sea salt, for seasoning
- Freshly ground black pepper, for seasoning
- 2 tablespoons fresh parsley, for garnish

Directions:

1. Using a large skillet, pour olive oil, then put it on a medium-high heat.

2. Sauté the onion and garlic until softened, about 3 minutes.

3. Add the tomatoes, edamame, corn, and bell pepper.

4. Make sure it boils, then reduce the heat to low and simmer until the vegetables are tender, about 15 minutes.

5. Season with salt and pepper.

6. Serve topped with parsley.

Nutrition: Calories: 265 Total Fat: 12g Protein: 11g Cholesterol: 0mg Sodium: 101mg Carbohydrates: 27g Fiber: 6g

31. Black-Eyed Pea Kale Bowl

Preparation Time: 10 minutes

Cooking Time: 20 minutes

Servings: 4

Ingredients:

- ½ cup brown rice
- 1 tablespoon olive oil
- ½ sweet onion, finely chopped
- 2 teaspoons minced garlic
- 2 (15-ounce) cans black peas
- 4 cups fresh kale
- 2 large tomatoes, finely chopped
- 3 tablespoons finely chopped chives

Directions:

1. Cook the rice and set aside. You can do this up to 3 days ahead, storing the rice in a sealed container in the refrigerator.

2. Pour on olive oil in a skillet and set it on medium-high heat.

3. Sauté the onion and garlic until softened, about 3 minutes.

4. Stir in the black-eyed peas and rice and cook until heated through, about 10 minutes.

5. Stir in the kale and sauté until wilted for five minutes.

6. Distribute mixture into 4 bowls and divide tomatoes between the bowls.

7. Serve topped with chives.

Nutrition: Calories: 257 Total Fat: 6g Protein: 13g Cholesterol: 0mg Sodium: 73mg Carbohydrates: 42g Fiber: 10g

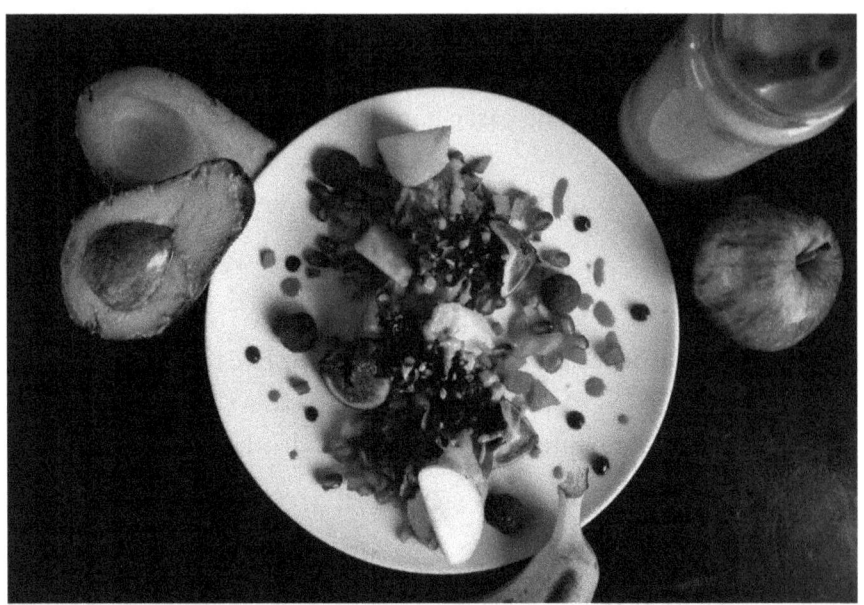

CHAPTER 7:

JUICES AND SMOOTHIES RECIPES

32. Groovy Green Smoothie

Preparation Time: 10 minutes

Cooking Time: 0 minutes

Servings: 2

Ingredients:

- 1 banana, cut in chunks
- 1 cup grapes
- 1 (6 ounces) tub vanilla yogurt
- 1/2 apple, cored and chopped

- 1 1/2 cups fresh spinach leaves

Directions:

1. Put the banana, grapes, yogurt, apple, and spinach in a blender. Cover and mix until smooth.

2. Pour into glasses and serve.

Nutrition: Calories 205 Fat 1.9g Carbohydrates 45g Protein 6.1g Cholesterol 4mg Sodium 76mg

33. Sun Juice

Preparation Time: 10 minutes

Cooking Time: 0 minutes

Servings: 1

Ingredients:

- 2 oranges, peeled and sliced
- 1/2 cup fresh raspberries
- 1 medium-sized banana, peeled
- 3 fresh mint leaves

Directions:

1. Juice everything in the juice machine. Pour on the ice to serve.

Nutrition: Calories 293 Fat 1.1g Carbohydrates 73.6g Protein 5g Cholesterol 0mg

34. Protein-Packed Blueberry Smoothie

Preparation Time: 5 minutes

Cooking Time: 0 minutes

Servings: 2

Ingredients:

- ¾ unsweetened coconut milk
- ½ cup unsweetened almond milk
- ⅓ Cup frozen blueberries
- 4 tablespoons vanilla protein powder

Directions:

1. Put everything into the blender until a smooth consistency is achieved. Serve and enjoy!

Nutrition: Fat: 6.1g Carbohydrates: 6g Protein: 6.4g

35. Strawberry Protein Smoothie

Preparation Time: 5 minutes

Cooking Time: 0 minutes

Servings: 2

Ingredients:

- ½ cup frozen strawberries

- 1 tablespoon almond butter

- ½ scoop vanilla protein powder

- ⅓ Cup almond milk

- ½ cup ice

Directions:

1. Put everything into the blender. Serve and enjoy!

Nutrition: Fat: 14.2g Carbohydrates: 7.5g Protein: 8.4g

36. Raspberry Avocado Smoothie

Preparation Time: 5 minutes

Cooking Time: 0 minutes

Servings: 2

Ingredients:

- 1 small ripe avocado, peeled and pitted
- ¼ cup raspberries, frozen
- 2 tablespoons lemon juice
- 1 cup water

Directions:

1. Put everything into the blender until a smooth consistency is achieved. Serve and enjoy!

Nutrition: Fat: 19.8g Carbohydrates: 10.8g Protein: 2.2g

37. Easy Antioxidant Smoothie

Preparation Time: 3 minutes

Cooking Time: 0 minutes

Servings: 2

Ingredients:

- 2-3 frozen broccoli florets
- 1 cup orange juice
- 2 plums, cut
- 1 cup raspberries
- 1 tsp. ginger powder

Directions:

1. Combine all ingredients in a high-speed blender and blend until smooth.

Nutrition: Calories: 150 Carbohydrates: 36g Total fat: 1g Protein: 1g

CHAPTER 8:

OTHER RECIPES

38. Black Beans & Brown Rice

Preparation Time: 2 Minutes

Cook Time: 45 Minutes

Servings: 4

Ingredients:

- 4 cups water
- 2 cups brown rice, uncooked
- 1 can no-salt black beans
- 3 cloves garlic, minced

Directions:

1. Bring the water and rice to boil, simmer for 40 minutes.

2. In a pan, cook the black beans with their liquid and the garlic for 5 minutes.

3. Toss the rice and beans together, and serve.

Nutrition: Calories 429 Fat 3.3g Carbohydrate 87.3g Protein 12.5g

39. Beans & Greens Bowl

Preparation Time: 2 Minutes

Cook Time: 2 Minutes

Servings: 1

Ingredients:

- 1½ cups curly kale, washed, chopped
- ½ cup black beans, cooked
- ½ avocado
- 2 Tbsps. feta cheese, crumbled

Directions:

1. Mix the kale and black beans in a microwavable bowl and heat for about 1 ½ minutes.
2. Add the avocado and stir well. Top with feta.

Nutrition: Calories 830 Fat 29.6g Carbohydrate 113.7g Protein 46.9g

40. Millet and Teff with Squash & Onions

Preparation Time: 10 Minutes Cook Time: 20 Minutes

Servings: 6

Ingredients:

- 1 cup millet
- ½ cup teff grain
- 4½ cups of water
- 1 onion, sliced
- 1 butternut squash, chopped
- ¼ tsp. Sea salt

Directions:

1. Rinse millet and put in a large pot.
2. Add remaining ingredients. Mix well.
3. Simmer 20 minutes until all the water is absorbed.
4. Serve hot.

Nutrition: Calories 218 Fat 1.7g Carbohydrate 45.2g Protein 6.6g

41. Quesadilla with Black Beans and Sweet Potato

Preparation Time: 10 minutes

Cook Time: 30 minutes

Servings: 2

Ingredients:

- 1 medium-sized sweet potato, peeled and cut into cubes
- 3 teaspoons taco seasoning
- 4 whole-wheat tortillas
- ½ of a 15-ounce can of black beans, drained and rinsed

Directions:

1. Bring a large pot of water to boil and drop in the sweet potato.
2. Boil for 10 to 20 minutes or until soft.
3. Drain the sweet potato and put it in a bowl.
4. Add the taco seasoning and mash well.
5. To assemble the quesadilla, spread the sweet potato mixture on the tortilla.
6. Add the black beans and press them into the potato mixture.

7. Cover with another tortilla.

8. Heat a nonstick skillet over medium-high heat and lay the tortilla in it. Toast on both sides and serve immediately.

Nutrition: Calories 520 Fat 3g Carbohydrate 99.8g Protein 26.9g

42. Meatless Chick Nuggets

Preparation Time: 10 minutes

Cook Time: 30 minutes

Servings: 8

Ingredients:

- 1 15.5-ounce can chickpeas, rinsed and drained
- ½ teaspoon garlic powder
- 1 teaspoon granulated onion
- 1 tablespoon nutritional yeast
- 1 tablespoon whole-wheat bread crumbs
- ½ cup panko bread crumbs

Directions:

1. Preheat the oven to 350 degrees Fahrenheit and cover a rimmed baking pan with parchment paper.
2. Place the drained chickpeas in a food processor and pulse four to five times.

3. Add the garlic powder, granulated onion, nutritional yeast, and the tablespoon of whole-wheat bread crumbs to the processor and process until you get a chunky, grainy mixture that sticks together.

4. Scoop out by teaspoonfuls and form balls.

5. Roll the balls in the panko crumbs and set them on the baking sheet, flattening each ball, so it looks more like a chicken nugget. Be sure to space them apart, so they do not touch each other.

6. Bake for 20 minutes, remove from the oven, and flip each nugget over with tongs. Return to the oven for 10 more minutes.

7. Cool for a few minutes, and then serve with honey, barbecue sauce, or Ranch dipping sauce.

Nutrition: Calories 245 Fat 4.4g Carbohydrate 41.6g Protein 12.5g

43. Apple Mint Salad with Pine Nut Crunch

Preparation Time: 10 Minutes

Cook Time: 0 Minutes

Servings: 2

Ingredients:

- 1 medium apple, diced
- 1 tablespoon lemon juice
- 1 teaspoon maple syrup
- ½ teaspoon dried mint
- 1 tablespoon fresh pomegranate seeds
- 1 teaspoon pine nuts or sliced almonds

Directions:

1. Toast the nuts in a pan on the stove. Stir constantly so they don't burn and let them turn a golden brown. Set the pan aside until cooled to room temperature.

2. Place the diced apple in a small bowl with the lemon juice and stir around, so all the apple is coated.

3. Add the maple syrup and dried mint and stir it in.

4. Sprinkle the top of the salad with pomegranate seeds and toasted nuts.

Nutrition: Calories 128 Fat 1.3g Carbohydrate 30g Protein 1.1g

44. Pleasant Lemonade

Time: 10 Minutes Cooking Time: 3 hours and 15 minutes

Servings: 10

Ingredients:

- Cinnamon sticks for serving

- 2 cups of coconut sugar

- 1/4 cup of honey

- 3 cups of lemon juice. Fresh

- 32 fluid ounce of water

Directions:

1. Using a 4-quarts slow cooker, place all the ingredients except for the cinnamon sticks and stir properly.

2. Cover it with the lid, then plug in the slow cooker and cook it for 3 hours on the low heat setting or until it is heated thoroughly. When done, stir properly and serve with the cinnamon sticks.

Nutrition: Calories: 146 Carbohydrates: 34g Protein: 0g Fats: 0g

45. Soothing Ginger Tea Drink

Preparation Time: 10 Minutes

Cooking Time: 2 hours and 15 minutes

Servings: 8

Ingredients:

- 1 tablespoon of minced gingerroot
- 2 tablespoons of honey
- 15 green tea bags
- 32 fluid ounce of white grape juice
- 2 quarts of boiling water

Directions:

1. Pour water into a 4-quarts slow cooker, immerse tea bags, cover the cooker, and let stand for 10 minutes.
2. After 10 minutes, remove and discard tea bags and stir in the remaining ingredients.
3. Return cover to slow cooker, then plug in and let cook at high heat setting for 2 hours or until heated through.

4. When done, strain the liquid and serve hot or cold.

Nutrition: Calories: 45 Carbohydrates: 12g Protein: 0g Fats: 0g

46. Nice Spiced Cherry Cider

Preparation Time: 10 Minutes

Cooking Time: 4 hours and 5 minutes

Servings: 16

Ingredients:

- 2 cinnamon sticks, each about 3 inches long
- 6-ounce of cherry gelatin
- 4 quarts of apple cider

Directions:

1. Using a 6-quarts slow cooker, pour the apple cider and add the cinnamon stick.

2. Stir, then cover the slow cooker with its lid. Plug in the cooker and let it cook for 3 hours at the high heat setting or until it is heated thoroughly.

3. Then add and stir the gelatin properly, then continue cooking for another hour.

4. When done, remove the cinnamon sticks and serve the drink hot or cold.

Nutrition: Calories: 100 Carbohydrates: 0g Protein: 0g Fats: 0g

47. Fragrant Spiced Coffee

Preparation Time: 10 Minutes

Cooking Time: 2 hours and 10 minutes

Servings: 8

Ingredients:

- 4 cinnamon sticks, each about 3 inches long
- 1 1/2 teaspoons of whole cloves
- 1/3 cup of honey
- 2-ounce of chocolate syrup
- 1/2 teaspoon of anise extract
- 8 cups of brewed coffee

Directions:

1. Pour the coffee into a 4-quarts slow cooker and pour in the remaining ingredients except for cinnamon and stir properly.
2. Wrap the whole cloves in cheesecloth and tie its corners with strings.

3. Immerse this cheesecloth bag in the liquid present in the slow cooker and cover it with the lid.

4. Then plug in the slow cooker and let it cook on the low heat setting for 3 hours or until heated thoroughly.

5. When done, discard the cheesecloth bag and serve.

Nutrition: Calories: 150 Carbohydrates: 35g Protein: 3g Fats: 0g

48. Banana Chips

Preparation Time: 15 Minutes

Cooking Time: 1 hour

Servings: 4

Ingredients:

- 2 large bananas, peeled and cut into ¼-inch thick slices
- ½ teaspoon ground cinnamon

Directions:

1. Prepare the oven to 250 degrees F. Line a large baking sheet with a parchment paper.
2. Place the banana slices onto a prepared baking sheet.
3. Bake for about 1 hour.
4. Remove from the oven and set aside to cool before serving.

Nutrition: Calories: 61 Fats: 0.2g Carbs: 15.8g Proteins: 0.8g

49. Dehydrated Oranges

Preparation Time: 10 Minutes

Cooking Time: 10 hours

Servings: 4

Ingredients:

- 2 seedless navel oranges, sliced thinly
- Salt, as required

Directions:

1. Set the dehydrator to 135 degrees F.
2. Arrange the orange slices onto the dehydrator sheets.
3. Dehydrate for about 10 hours.
4. Remove the orange slices from the dehydrator and set aside to cool completely before serving.

Nutrition: Calories: 43 Fats: 0.1g Carbs: 10.8g Proteins: 0.9g

50. Sweet Potato Mash

Preparation Time: 15 Minutes

Cooking Time: 20 minutes

Servings: 4

Ingredients:

- 3 medium sweet potatoes, peeled and cut into 2-inch chunks
- ¼ cup unsweetened almond milk
- 1-2 tablespoons maple syrup
- Salt, as required
- ¼ teaspoon ground cinnamon
- Pinch of ground nutmeg

Directions:

1. In a large pan of boiling water, arrange a steamer basket.
2. Place the sweet potato chunks in the steamer basket.
3. Cover and steam for about 15-20 minutes or until desired doneness.
4. Drain well and transfer the sweet potato chunks into a bowl.

5. With a potato masher, mash the chunks.

6. Add the remaining ingredients and mix until well combined.

7. Serve immediately.

Nutrition: Calories: 142 Fats: 0.4g Carbs: 33.2g Proteins: 1.7g

CONCLUSION

Well done! Thank you for reaching the end of this book, The Complete Vegetarian Cookbook.

Hopefully, this book has helped you understand that making vegetarian recipes and diet easier can improve your life, not only by improving your health and helping you lose weight, but also by saving you money and time.

Remember that vegetarianism is a choice, not a religion.

Be flexible when it comes to your diet and enjoy new tastes and experiences.

Don't be afraid of meat substitutes, but experiment with using them sparingly. There is no need to completely replace meat with fake meat products like tofu or processed soy-based vegetarian burgers and hot dogs. Not only are they expensive, but fake meats contain artificial ingredients that may or may not be healthy for you.

Also, if you are not used to eating a vegetarian diet, start with a few vegetarian meals and snacks during the week, and see how you feel.

You can always add more vegetarian meals to your diet later. It is better to be even slightly vegetarians than completely non-vegetarian.

The best tip I can give you about making vegetarian recipes is to experiment and have fun!

Here are some more tips to help you with your vegetarian diet:

1. Remember that vegetarianism is not a destination, it is a journey.

2. A vegetarian diet is plant-based. This means that you should try to eat more plants and less animal products. You should also be careful not to replace whole foods with their processed counterparts, such as replacing whole foods such as fruits and vegetables with fruit juice and pasta sauce.

3. Try to avoid processed food whenever possible, while still maintaining your balanced diet and nutrients that you need for your health. An easier way of doing this will be to make your own food when

possible and try to avoid packaged, pre-prepared foods at the grocery store.

4. Avoid processed food products that contain artificial ingredients, such as sweeteners, colors, and flavors.

5. Avoid highly processed meat substitutes. Remember to use meat substitutes in moderation or as an occasional treat.

6. If you choose to eat meat substitutes such as tofu, be sure to thoroughly cook it and try different ways of preparing it

7. You may need to gradually introduce your family and friends to your new eating habits. Don't expect everyone to support you or enjoy the same things you do when it comes to vegetarian recipes. As long as you are happy with your food choices, that is the most important thing – even if it means making some changes at home!

When you are having a hard time, always remember this: You can always choose to stop being a vegetarian.

You can simply start eating meat again if you are struggling with your new diet.

Remember that it is okay to be a part-time vegetarian, but if you find that you cannot maintain the lifestyle or are unhappy with your choice, it is always better to go back to eating a non-veg diet.

There is no shame in making changes to your vegetarian recipe routine if you need to, and you will not shame yourself for deciding that a strict vegetarian diet does not work for you.

I know that there are many books and choosing my book is amazing. I am thankful that you stopped and took the time to decide. You made a great decision, and I am sure that you enjoyed it.

I will be even happier if you will add some comments. Feedbacks helped by growing, and they still do. They help me to choose better content and new ideas. So, maybe your feedback can trigger an idea for my next book. Thank you again for downloading this book!

I hope you enjoyed reading my book!

www.ingramcontent.com/pod-product-compliance
Lightning Source LLC
Chambersburg PA
CBHW070724030426
42336CB00013B/1911